The Ult

Cookbook

The tasty easy and delicious vegan recipes to stay healthy. Easy meals to start a healthy diet without meat.

Helena Owen

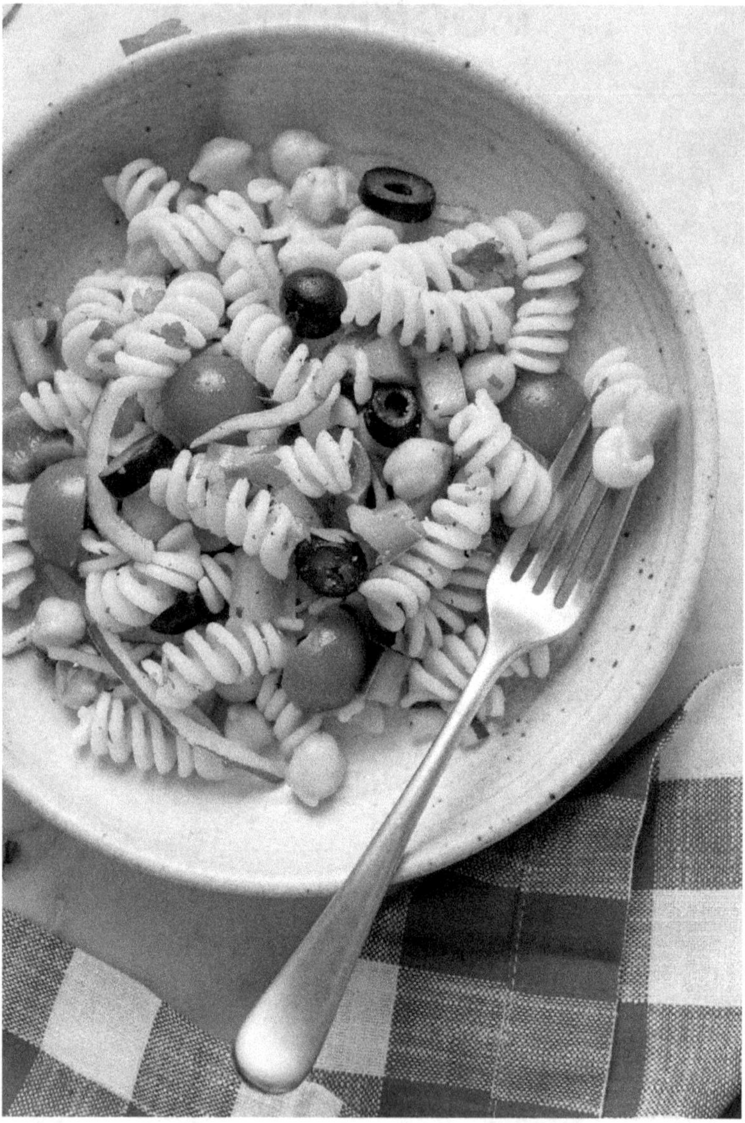

Table of Contents

INTRODUCTION

The Merriam Webster Dictionary defines a vegetarian as one contains a wholly of vegetables, grains, nuts, fruits, and sometimes eggs or dairy products. It has also been described as a plant-based diet that relies wholly on plant-foods such as fruits, whole grains, herbs, vegetables, nuts, seeds, and spices. Whatever way you want to look at it, the reliance wholly on plants stands the vegetarian diet out from other types of diets. People become vegetarians for different reasons. Some take up this nutritional plan for medical or health reasons. For example, people suffering from cardiovascular diseases or who stand the risk of developing such diseases are usually advised to refrain from meat generally and focus on a plant-based diet, rich in fruits and vegetables. Some other individuals become vegetarians for religious or ethical reasons.

On this side of the spectrum are Hinduism, Jainism, Buddhism, Seventh-Day Adventists, and some other religions. It is believed that being a vegetarian is part of being holy and keeping with the ideals of non-violence. For ethical reasons, some animal rights activists are also vegetarians based on the belief that animals have rights and should not be slaughtered for food. Yet another set of persons become vegetarians based on food preference. Such individuals are naturally more disposed to a plant-based diet and find meat and other related food products less pleasurable. Some refrain from meat as a protest against climate change. This is based on the environmental concern that rearing livestock contributes to climate change and greenhouse gas emissions and the waste of natural resources in maintaining such livestock. People are usually very quick to throw words around without exactly knowing what a Vegetarian Diet means. In the same vein, the term "vegetarian" has become a popular one in recent years. What exactly does this word connote, and what does it not mean?

At its simplest, the word "vegetarian" refers to a person who refrains from eating meat, beef, pork, lard, chicken, or even fish. Depending on the kind of vegetarian it is, however, a vegetarian could either eat or exclude from his diet animal products. Animal products would refer to foods such as eggs, dairy products, and even honey! A vegetarian diet would, therefore, refer to the nutritional plan of the void of meat. It is the eating lifestyle of individuals who depend on plant-based foods for nutrition. It excludes animal products, particularly meat - a common denominator for all kinds of Vegetarians - from their diets. A vegetarian could also be defined as a meal plan that consists of foods coming majorly from plants to the exclusion of meat, poultry, and seafood.

This kind of Vegetarian diet usually contains no animal protein.

It is completely understandable from the discussion so far that the term "vegetarian" is more or less a blanket term covering different plant-based diets. While reliance majorly on plant foods is consistent in all the different types of vegetarians, they have some underlying differences. The different types of vegetarians are discussed below:

Veganism: This is undoubtedly the strictest type of vegetarian diet. Vegans exclude the any animal product. It goes as far as avoiding animal-derived ingredients contained in processed foods. Whether its meat, poultry products like eggs, dairy products inclusive of milk, honey, or even gelatin, they all are excluded from the vegans.

Some vegans go beyond nutrition and go as far as refusing to wear clothes that contain animal products. This means such vegans do not wear leather, wool, or silk.

Lacto-vegetarian: This kind of vegetarian excludes meat, fish, and poultry. However, it allows the inclusion of dairy products such as milk, yogurt, cheese, and butter. The hint is perhaps in the name since Lacto means milk in Latin.

Ovo-Vegetarian: Meat and dairy products are excluded under this diet, but eggs could be consumed. Ovo means egg.

Lacto-Ovo Vegetarian: This appears to be the hybrid of the Ovo Vegetarian and the Lacto-Vegetarian. This is the most famous type of vegetarian diet and is usually what comes to mind when people think of the Vegetarian. This type of Vegetarian bars all kinds of meat but allows for the consumption of eggs and dairy products.

Pollotarian: This vegetarian allows the consumption of chicken.

Pescatarian: This refers to the vegetarian that consumes fish. More people are beginning to subscribe to this kind of diet due to health reasons.

Flexitarian: Flexitarians are individuals who prefer plant-based foods to meat but have no problem eating meats once in a while. They are also referred to as semi-vegetarians.

Raw Vegan: This is also called the raw food and consists of a vegan that is yet to be processed and has also not been heated over 46 C. This kind of diet has its root in the belief that nutrients and minerals present in the plant diet are lost when cooked on temperature above 46 C and could also become harmful to the body.

STIR-FRIED, GRILLED VEGETABLES

Crusty Grilled Corn

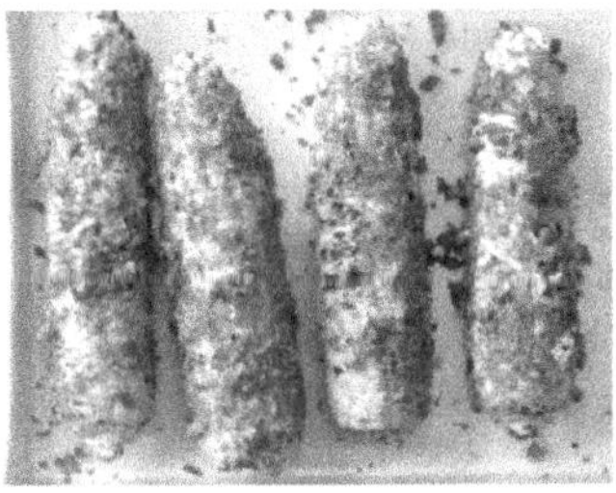

Preparation Time: 10 minutes

Cooking Time: 15 minutes

Servings: 4

Ingredients:

- 2 corn cobs
- 1/3 cup Vegenaise
- 1 small handful cilantro
- ½ cup breadcrumbs
- 1 teaspoon lemon juice

Directions:

1. Preheat the gas grill on high heat.

2. Add corn grill to the grill and continue grilling until it turns golden-brown on all sides.
3. Mix the Vegenaise, cilantro, breadcrumbs, and lemon juice in a bowl.
4. Add grilled corn cobs to the crumbs mixture.
5. Toss well then serve.

Nutrition: Calories: 253 Total Fat: 13g Protein: 31g Total Carbs: 3g Fiber: 0g Net Carbs: 3g

Grilled Carrots with Chickpea Salad

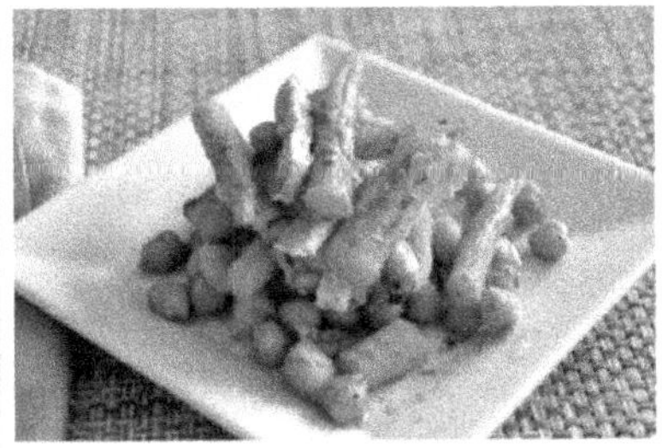

Preparation Time: 10 minutes

Cooking Time: 10 minutes

Servings: 8

Ingredients:

- Carrots
- 8 large carrots
- 1 tablespoon oil
- 1 ½ teaspoon salt
- 1 teaspoon dried oregano
- 1 teaspoon dried thyme
- 2 teaspoon paprika powder
- 1 ½ tablespoon soy sauce
- ½ cup of water
- Chickpea Salad
- 14 oz. canned chickpeas

- 3 medium pickles
- 1 small onion
- A big handful of lettuce
- 1 teaspoon apple cider vinegar
- ½ teaspoon dried oregano
- ½ teaspoon salt
- Ground black pepper, to taste
- ½ cup vegan cream

Directions:

1. Toss the carrots with all of its ingredients in a bowl.
2. Thread one carrot on a stick and place it on a plate.
3. Preheat the grill over high heat.
4. Grill the carrots for 2 minutes per side on the grill.
5. Toss the ingredients for the salad in a large salad bowl.
6. Slice grilled carrots and add them on top of the salad.
7. Serve fresh.

Nutrition: Calories: 661 Total Fat: 68g Carbs: 17g Net Carbs: 7g Fiber: 2g Protein: 4g

Grilled Avocado Guacamole

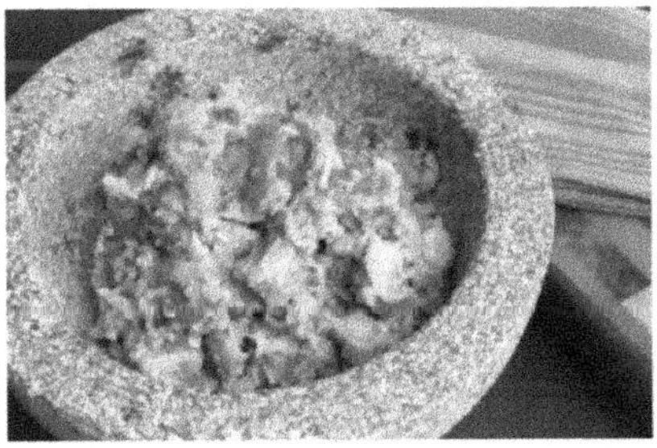

Preparation Time: 10 minutes

Cooking Time: 20 minutes

Servings: 4

Ingredients:

- ½ teaspoon olive oil
- 1 lime, halved
- ½ onion, halved
- 1 serrano chile, halved, stemmed, and seeded
- 3 Haas avocados, skin on
- 2–3 tablespoons fresh cilantro, chopped
- ½ teaspoon smoked salt

Directions:

1. Preheat the grill over medium heat.
2. Brush the grilling grates with olive oil and place chile, onion, and lime on it.

3. Grill the onion for 10 minutes, chile for 5 minutes, and lime for 2 minutes.
4. Transfer the veggies to a large bowl.
5. Now cut the avocados in half and grill them for 5 minutes.
6. Mash the flesh of the grilled avocado in a bowl.
7. Chop the other grilled veggies and add them to the avocado mash.
8. Stir in remaining ingredients and mix well.
9. Serve.

Nutrition: Calories: 165 Total Fat: 17g Carbs: 4g Net Carbs: 2g Fiber: 1g Protein: 1g

Grilled Fajitas with Jalapeño Sauce

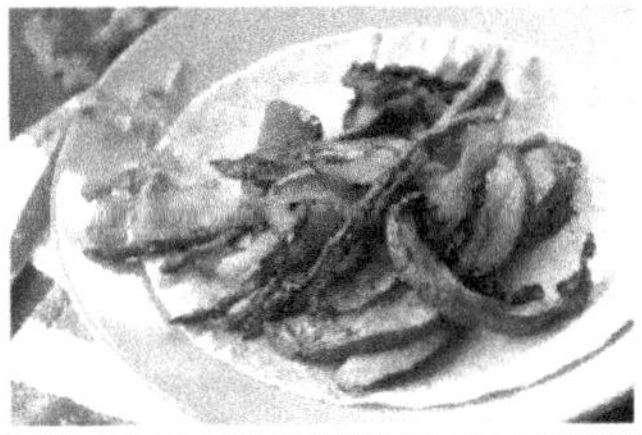

Preparation Time: 10 minutes

Cooking Time: 25 minutes

Servings: 4

Ingredients:

- Marinade
- ¼ cup olive oil
- ¼ cup lime juice
- 2 garlic cloves, minced
- 1 teaspoon chili powder
- 1 teaspoon ground cumin
- 1 teaspoon dried oregano
- ½ teaspoon salt
- ½ teaspoon black pepper
- Jalapeño Sauce
- 6 jalapeno peppers stemmed, halved, and seeded

- 1–2 teaspoons olive oil
- 1 cup raw cashews, soaked and drained
- ½ cup almond milk
- ¼ cup water
- ¼ cup lime juice
- 2 teaspoons agaves
- ½ cup fresh cilantro
- Salt, to taste
- Grilled Vegetables
- ½ lb. asparagus spears, trimmed
- 2 large portobello mushrooms, sliced
- 1 large zucchini, sliced
- 1 red bell pepper, sliced
- 1 red onion, sliced

Directions:

1. Dump all the ingredients for the marinade in a large bowl.
2. Toss in all the veggies and mix well to marinate for 1 hour.
3. Meanwhile, prepare the sauce and brush the jalapenos with oil.
4. Grill the jalapenos for 5 minutes per side until slightly charred.

5. Blend the grilled jalapenos with other ingredients for the sauce in a blender.
6. Transfer this sauce to a separate bowl and keep it aside.
7. Now grill the marinated veggies in the grill until soft and slightly charred on all sides.
8. Pour the prepared sauce over the grilled veggies.
9. Serve.

Nutrition: Calories: 663 Total Fat: 68g Carbs: 20g Net Carbs: 10g Fiber: 2g Protein: 4g

Grilled Ratatouille Kebabs

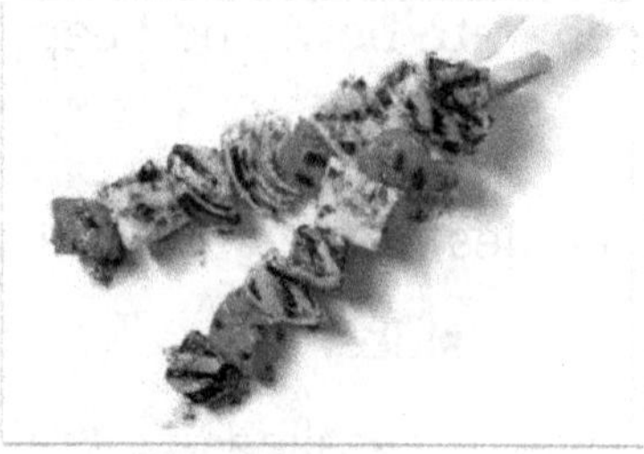

Preparation Time: 10 minutes

Cooking Time: 20 minutes

Servings: 6

Ingredients:

- 3 tablespoons soy sauce
- 3 tablespoons balsamic vinegar
- 1 teaspoon dried thyme leaves
- 2 tablespoons extra virgin olive oil
- Veggies
- 1 zucchini, diced
- ½ red onion, diced
- ½ red capsicum, diced
- 2 tomatoes, diced
- 1 small eggplant, diced
- 8 button mushrooms, diced

Directions:

1. Toss the veggies with soy sauce, olive oil, thyme, and balsamic vinegar in a large bowl.
2. Thread the veggies alternately on the wooden skewers and reserve the remaining marinade.
3. Marinate these skewers for 1 hour in the refrigerator.
4. Preheat the grill over medium heat.
5. Grill the marinated skewers for 5 minutes per side while basting with the reserved marinade.
6. Serve fresh.

Nutrition: Calories: 166 Total Fat: 17g Carbs: 5g Net Carbs: 3g Fiber: 1g Protein: 1g

Tofu Hoagie Rolls

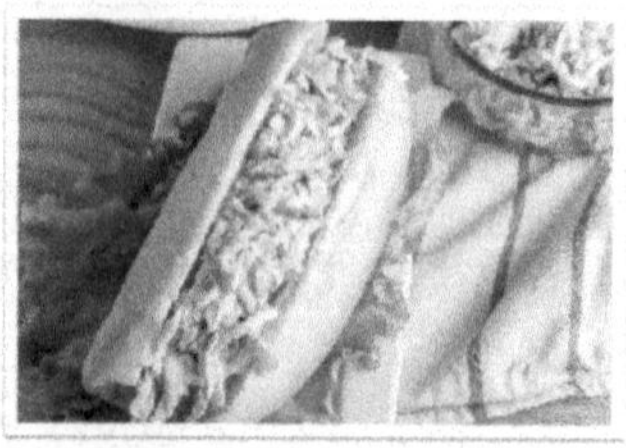

Preparation Time: 10 minutes

Cooking Time: 20 minutes

Servings: 6

Ingredients:

- ½ cup vegetable broth
- ¼ cup hot sauce
- 1 tablespoon vegan butter
- 1 (16 ounce) package tofu, pressed and diced
- 4 cups cabbage, shredded
- 2 medium apples, grated
- 1 medium shallot, grated
- 6 tablespoons vegan mayonnaise
- 1 tablespoon apple cider vinegar
- Salt and black pepper
- 4 6-inch hoagie rolls, toasted

Directions:

1. In a saucepan, combine broth with butter and hot sauce and bring to a boil.
2. Add tofu and reduce the heat to a simmer.
3. Cook for 10 minutes then remove from heat and let sit for 10 minutes to marinate.
4. Toss cabbage and rest of the ingredients in a salad bowl.
5. Prepare and set up a grill on medium heat.
6. Drain the tofu and grill for 5 minutes per side.
7. Lay out the toasted hoagie rolls and add grilled tofu to each hoagie
8. Add the cabbage mixture evenly between them then close it.
9. Serve.

Nutrition: Calories: 111 Total Fat: 11g Carbs: 5g Net Carbs: 1g Fiber: 0g Protein: 1g

Grilled Avocado with Tomatoes

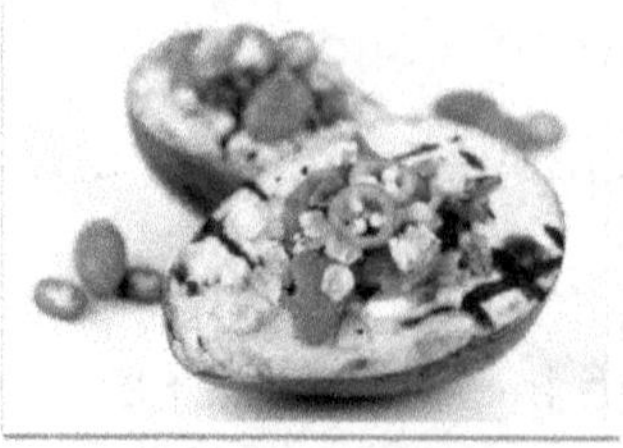

Preparation Time: 10 minutes

Cooking Time: 15 minutes

Servings: 6

Ingredients:

- 3 avocados, halved and pitted
- 3 limes, wedged
- 1½ cup grape tomatoes
- 1 cup fresh corn
- 1 cup onion, chopped
- 3 serrano peppers
- 2 garlic cloves, peeled
- ¼ cup cilantro leaves, chopped
- 1 tablespoon olive oil
- Salt and black pepper to taste

Directions:

1. Prepare and set a grill over medium heat.

2. Brush the avocado with oil and grill it for 5 minutes per side.
3. Meanwhile, toss the garlic, onion, corn, tomatoes, and pepper in a baking sheet.
4. At 550 degrees F, roast the vegetables for 5 minutes.
5. Toss the veggie mix and stir in salt, cilantro, and black pepper.
6. Mix well then fill the grilled avocadoes with the mixture.
7. Garnish with lime.
8. Serve.

Nutrition: Calories: 56 Total Fat: 6g Carbs: 3g Net Carbs: 1g Fiber: 0g Protein: 1g

Grilled Tofu with Chimichurri Sauce

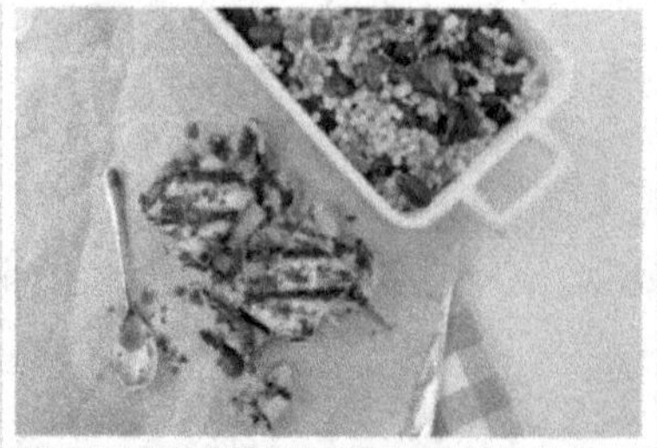

Preparation Time: 10 minutes

Cooking Time: 12 minutes

Servings: 4

Ingredients:

- 2 tablespoons plus 1 teaspoon olive oil
- 1 teaspoon dried oregano
- 1 cup parsley leaves
- ½ cup cilantro leaves
- 2 Fresno peppers, seeded and chopped
- 2 tablespoons white wine vinegar
- 2 tablespoons water
- 1 tablespoon fresh lime juice
- Salt and black pepper
- 1 cup couscous, cooked
- 1 teaspoon lime zest

- ¼ cup toasted pumpkin seeds
- 1 cup fresh spinach, chopped
- 1 (15.5 ounce) can kidney beans, rinsed and drained
- 1 (14 to 16 ounce) block tofu, diced
- 2 summer squashes, diced
- 3 spring onions, quartered

Directions:

1. In a saucepan, heat 2 tablespoons oil and add oregano over medium heat.
2. After 30 seconds add parsley, chili pepper, cilantro, lime juice, 2 tablespoons water, vinegar, salt and black pepper.
3. Mix well then blend in a blender.
4. Add the remaining oil, pumpkin seeds, beans and spinach and cook for 3 minutes.
5. Stir in couscous and adjust seasoning with salt and black pepper.
6. Prepare and set up a grill on medium heat.
7. Thread the tofu, squash, and onions on the skewer in an alternating pattern.
8. Grill these skewers for 4 minutes per side while basting with the green sauce.

9. Serve the skewers on top of the couscous with green sauce.
10. Enjoy.

Nutrition: Calories: 813 Total Fat: 83g Carbs: 25g Net Carbs: 11g Fiber: 1g Protein: 7g

Grilled Seitan with Creole Sauce

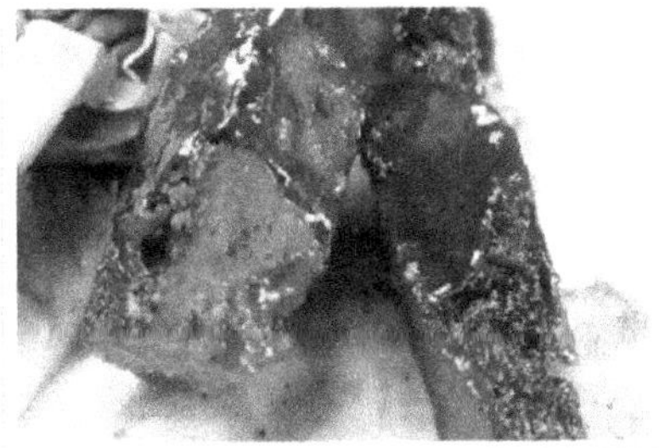

Preparation Time: 10 minutes

Cooking Time: 14 minutes

Servings: 4

Ingredients:

Grilled Seitan Kebabs:

- 4 cups seitan, diced
- 2 medium onions, diced into squares
- 8 bamboo skewers
- 1 can coconut milk
- 2½ tablespoons creole spice
- 2 tablespoons tomato paste
- 2 cloves of garlic

Creole Spice Mix:

- 2 tablespoons paprika
- 12 dried peri chili peppers
- 1 tablespoon salt

- 1 tablespoon freshly ground pepper
- 2 teaspoons dried thyme
- 2 teaspoons dried oregano

Directions:

1. Prepare the creole seasoning by blending all its ingredients and preserve in a sealable jar.
2. Thread seitan and onion on the bamboo skewers in an alternating pattern.
3. On a baking sheet, mix coconut milk with creole seasoning, tomato paste and garlic.
4. Soak the skewers in the milk marinade for 2 hours.
5. Prepare and set up a grill over medium heat.
6. Grill the skewers for 7 minutes per side.
7. Serve.

Nutrition: Calories: 407 Total Fat: 42g Carbs: 13gNet Carbs: 6g Fiber: 1g Protein: 4g

Mushroom Steaks

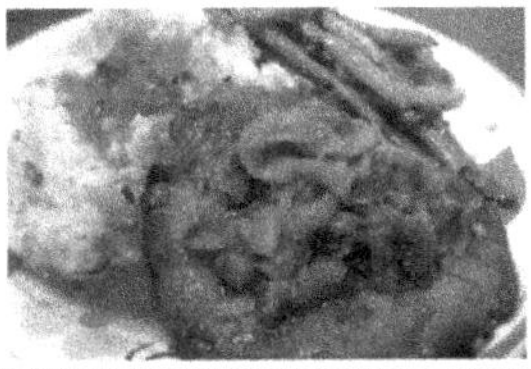

Preparation Time: 10 minutes

Cooking Time: 24 minutes

Servings: 4

Ingredients:

- 1 tablespoon vegan butter
- ½ cup vegetable broth
- ½ small yellow onion, diced
- 1 large garlic clove, minced
- 3 tablespoons balsamic vinegar
- 1 tablespoon mirin
- ½ tablespoon soy sauce
- ½ tablespoon tomato paste
- 1 teaspoon dried thyme
- ½ teaspoon dried basil
- A dash of ground black pepper
- 2 large, whole portobello mushrooms

Directions:

1. Melt butter in a saucepan over medium heat and stir in half of the broth.
2. Bring to a simmer then add garlic and onion. Cook for 8 minutes.
3. Whisk the rest of the ingredients except the mushrooms in a bowl.
4. Add this mixture to the onion in the pan and mix well.
5. Bring this filling to a simmer then remove from the heat.
6. Clean the mushroom caps inside and out and divide the filling between the mushrooms.
7. Place the mushrooms on a baking sheet and top them with remaining sauce and broth.
8. Cover with foil then place it on a grill to smoke.
9. Cover the grill and broil for 16 minutes over indirect heat.
10. Serve warm.

Nutrition: Calories: 887 Total Fat: 93g Carbs: 29g Net Carbs: 13g Fiber: 4g Protein: 8g

Zucchini Boats with Garlic Sauce

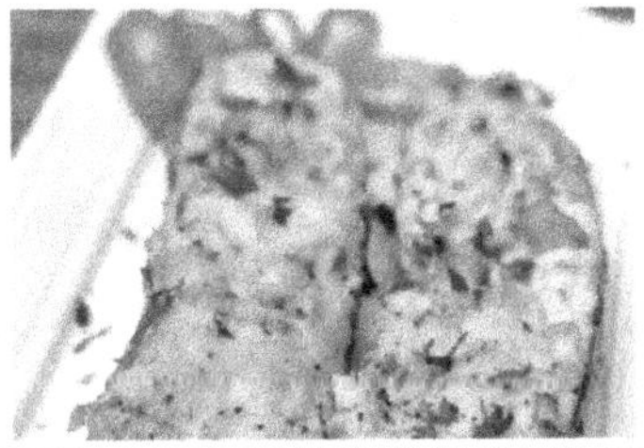

Preparation Time: 10 minutes

Cooking Time: 10 minutes

Servings: 2

Ingredients:

- 1 zucchini
- 1 tbsp. olive oil
- Salt, to taste
- Black pepper, to taste
- Filling:
- 1 cup organic walnuts
- 2 tablespoons olive oil
- ½ teaspoon smoked paprika
- ½ teaspoon ground cumin
- 1 pinch salt

Sauce:

- ½ cup cashews
- ½ cup water

- 2 teaspoons olive oil
- 2 teaspoons lemon juice
- 1 clove garlic
- 1/8 teaspoon salt

Directions:

- Cut the zucchini squash in half and scoop out some flesh from the center to make boats.
- Rub the zucchini boats with oil, salt, and black pepper.
- Prepare and set up a grill over medium heat.
- Grill the boats for 5 minutes per side.
- In a blender, add all the filling ingredients and blend them well.
- Divide the filling between the zucchini boats.
- Blend all of the sauce ingredients until it is lump free.
- Pour the sauce over the zucchini boats.
- Serve.

Nutrition: Calories: 444 Total Fat: 47g Carbs: 15g Net Carbs: 7g Fiber: 2g Protein: 4g

Grilled Eggplant with Pecan Butter Sauce

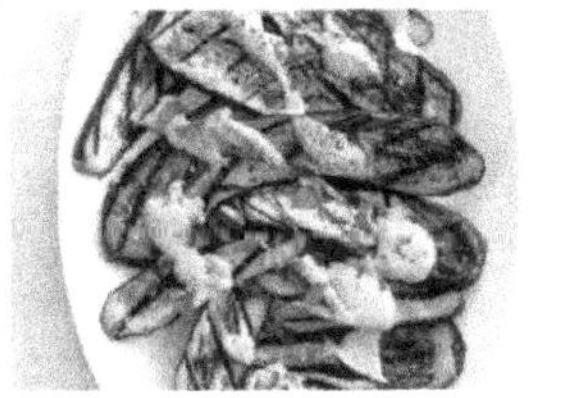

Preparation Time: 10 minutes

Cooking Time: 31 minutes

Servings: 02

Ingredients:

- Marinated Eggplant:
- 1 eggplant, sliced
- Salt to taste
- 4 tablespoons olive oil
- ¼ teaspoon smoked paprika
- ¼ teaspoon ground turmeric
- Black Bean and Pecan Sauce:
- 1/3 cup vegetable broth
- 1/3 cup red wine
- 1/3 cup red wine vinegar
- 1 large shallot, chopped
- 1 teaspoon ground coriander

- 2 teaspoons minced cilantro
- ½ cup pecan pieces, toasted
- 2 roasted garlic cloves
- 4 small banana peppers, seeded, and diced
- 8 tablespoons butter
- 1 tablespoon chives, chopped
- 1 (15.5 ounce) can black beans, rinsed and drained
- Salt and black pepper to taste
- 1 teaspoon fresh lime juice

Directions:

1. In a saucepan, add broth, wine, vinegar, shallots, coriander, cilantro and garlic.
2. Cook while stirring for 20 minutes on a simmer.
3. Meanwhile blend butter with chives, pepper, and pecans in a blender.
4. Add this mixture to the broth along with salt, lime juice, black pepper, and beans.
5. Mix well and cook for 5 minutes.
6. Rub the eggplant with salt and spices.
7. Prepare and set up the grill over medium heat.
8. Grill the eggplant slices for 6 minutes per side.
9. Serve the eggplant with prepared sauce.
10. Enjoy.

Nutrition: Calories: 441 Total Fat: 42g Carbs: 21g Net Carbs: 8g Fiber: 1g Protein: 7g

Sweet Potato Grilled Sandwich

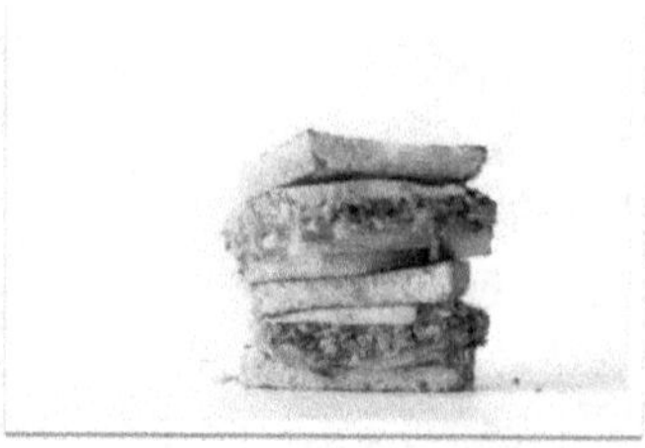

Preparation Time: 10 minutes

Cooking Time: 12 minutes

Servings: 2

Ingredients:

- 1 small sweet potato, sliced
- ½ cup sweet bell peppers, sliced
- 1 cup canned black beans, roughly mashed
- ½ cup salsa
- 1 avocado, peeled and sliced
- 4 slices bread
- 1-2 tablespoons vegan butter

Directions:

1. Prepare and set up the grill over medium heat.
1. Grill the sweet potato slices for 5 minutes and the bell pepper slices for 3 minutes.
2. Spread each slice of bread liberally with butter.

3. On two of the bread slices, layer sweet potato slices, bell peppers, beans, salsa and avocado slices.
4. Place the other two slices of bread on top to make two sandwiches.
5. Cut them in half diagonally then grill the sandwiches for 1 minute per side.
6. Serve.

Nutrition: Calories: 221 Total Fat: 21g Carbs: 11g Net Carbs: 4g Fiber: 1g Protein: 4g

Grilled Eggplant

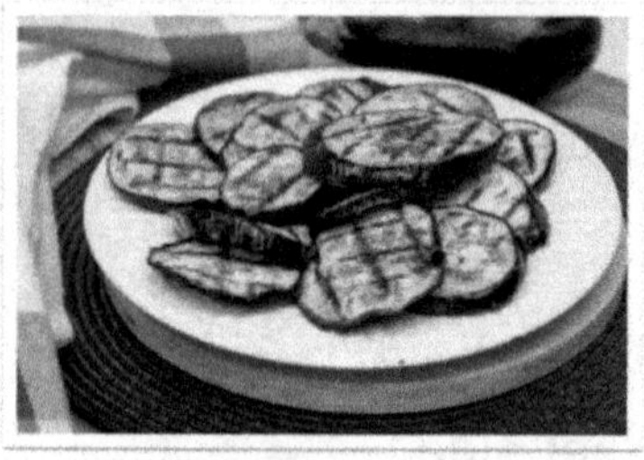

Preparation Time: 10 minutes

Cooking Time: 10 minutes

Servings: 04

Ingredients:

- 2 tablespoons salt
- 1 cup water
- 3 medium eggplants, sliced
- 1/3 cup olive oil

Directions:

1. Mix water with salt in a bowl and soak eggplants for 10 minutes.
2. Drain the eggplant and leave them in a colander.
3. Pat them dry with a paper towel.
4. Prepare and set up the grill at medium heat.
5. Toss the eggplant slices in olive oil.
6. Grill them for 5 minutes per side.
7. Serve.

Nutrition: Calories: 807 Total Fat: 85g Carbs: 15g Net Carbs: 7g Fiber: 1g Protein: 8g

Grilled Portobello

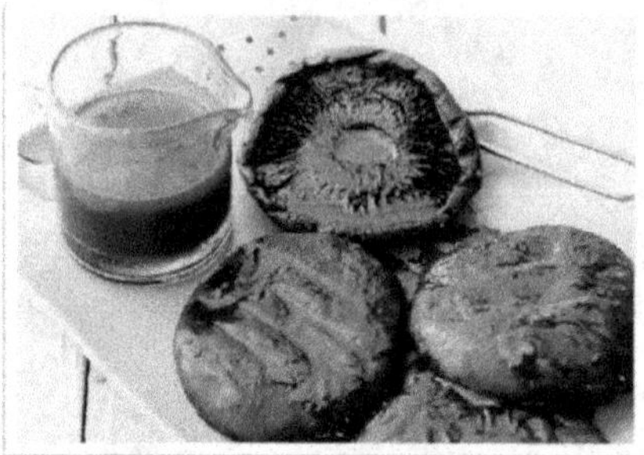

Preparation Time: 10 minutes

Cooking Time: 8 minutes

Servings: 04

Ingredients:

- 4 portobello mushrooms
- ¼ cup soy sauce
- ¼ cup tomato sauce
- 2 tablespoons maple syrup
- 1 tablespoon molasses
- 2 tablespoons minced garlic
- 1 tablespoon onion powder
- 1 pinch salt and pepper

Directions:

1. Mix all the ingredients except mushrooms in a bowl.

2. Add mushrooms to this marinade and mix well to coat.
3. Cover and marinate for 1 hour.
4. Prepare and set up the grill at medium heat. Grease it with cooking spray.
5. Grill the mushroom for 4 minutes per side.
6. Serve

Nutrition: Calories: 404 Total Fat: 43g Carbs: 8g Net Carbs: 4g Fiber: 1g Protein: 4g

Ginger Sweet Tofu

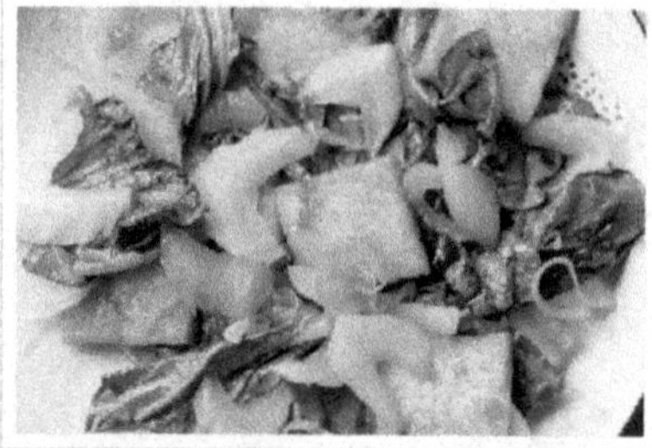

Preparation Time: 10 minutes

Cooking Time: 15 minutes

Servings: 04

Ingredients:

- ½ pound firm tofu, drained and diced
- 2 tablespoons peanut oil
- 1-inch piece ginger, sliced
- 1/3 pound bok choy, leaves separated
- 1 tablespoon shao sing rice wine
- 1 tablespoon rice vinegar
- ½ teaspoon dried chili flakes

Marinade:

- 1 tablespoon grated ginger
- 1 teaspoon dark soy sauce
- 2 tablespoons light soy sauce
- 1 tablespoon brown sugar

Directions:

1. Toss the tofu cubes with the marinade ingredients and marinate for 15 minutes.
2. In a wok, add half of the oil and ginger, then sauté for 30 secs.
3. Toss in bok choy and cook for 2 minutes.
4. Add a splash of water and steam for 2 minutes.
5. Transfer the bok choy to a bowl.
6. Add remaining oil and tofu to the pan then sauté for 10 minutes.
7. Add the tofu to the bok choy.
8. Serve.

Nutrition: Calories: 827 Total Fat: 85g Carbs: 17g Net Carbs: 7g Fiber: 2g Protein: 8g

Singapore Tofu

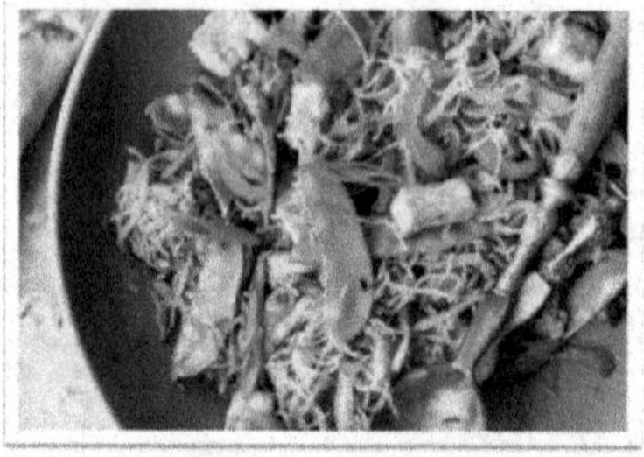

Preparation Time: 10 minutes

Cooking Time: 8 minutes

Servings: 04

Ingredients:

- ounces fine rice noodles, boiled
- 4 ounces firm tofu, boiled
- 2 tablespoons sunflower oil
- 3 spring onions, shredded
- 1 small piece of ginger, chopped
- 1 red pepper, thinly sliced
- ounces snap peas
- ounces beansprouts
- 1 teaspoon tikka masala paste
- 2 teaspoons reduced-salt soy sauce
- 1 tablespoon sweet chili sauce
- Chopped coriander and lime
- Lime wedges, to serve

Directions:

1. In a wok, add 1 tablespoon oil and the tofu then sauté for 5 minutes.
2. Transfer the sautéed tofu to a bowl.
3. Add more oil and the rest of the ingredients except noodles to the wok.
4. Stir fry for 3 minutes then add the tofu.
5. Toss well and then add noodles.
6. Mix and serve with lime wedges.

Nutrition: Calories: 414 Total Fat: 43g Carbs: 9g Net Carbs: 4g Fiber: 1g Protein: 4g

Wok Fried Broccoli

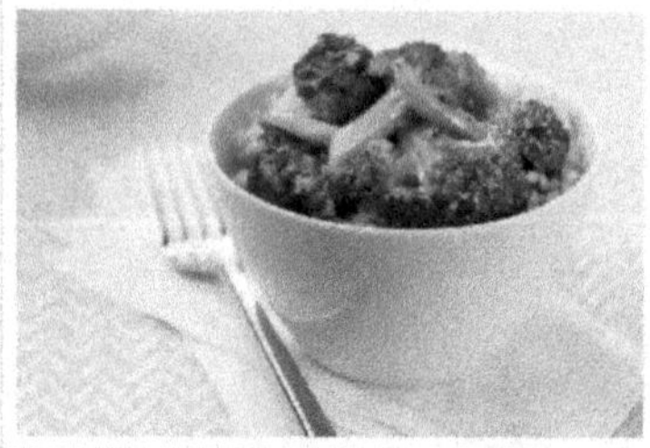

Preparation Time: 10 minutes

Cooking Time: 16 minutes

Servings: 02

Ingredients:

- 3 ounces whole, blanched peanuts
- 2 tablespoons olive oil
- 1 banana shallot, sliced
- 10 ounces broccoli, trimmed and cut into florets
- ¼ red pepper, julienned
- ½ yellow pepper, julienned
- 1 teaspoon soy sauce

Directions:

1. Toast peanuts on a baking sheet for 15 minutes at 350 degrees F.
2. In a wok, add oil and shallots and sauté for 10 minutes.
3. Toss in broccoli and peppers.

4. Stir fry for 3 minutes then add the rest of the ingredients.
5. Cook for 3 additional minutes and serve.

Nutrition: Calories: 391 Total Fat: 39g Carbs: 15g Net Carbs: 5g Fiber: 2g Protein: 6g

Broccoli & Brown Rice Satay

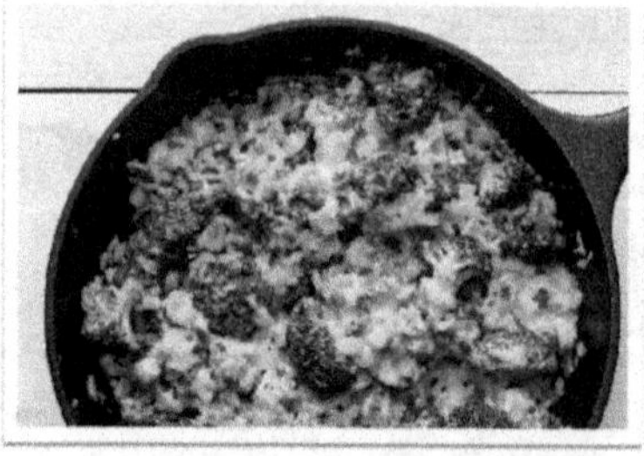

Preparation Time: 10 minutes

Cooking Time: 10 minutes

Servings: 4

Ingredients:

- 6 trimmed broccoli florets, halved
- 1-inch piece of ginger, shredded
- 2 garlic cloves, shredded
- 1 red onion, sliced
- 1 roasted red pepper, cut into cubes
- 2 teaspoons olive oil
- 1 teaspoon mild chili powder
- 1 tablespoon reduced salt soy sauce
- 1 tablespoon maple syrup
- 1 cup cooked brown rice

Directions:

1. Boil broccoli in water for 4 minutes then drain immediately.

2. In a pan add olive oil, ginger, onion, and garlic.
3. Stir fry for 2 minutes then add the rest of the ingredients.
4. Cook for 3 minutes then serve.

Nutrition: Calories: 196 Total Fat: 20g Carbs: 8g Net Carbs: 3g Fiber: 1g Protein: 3g

Sautéed Sesame Spinach

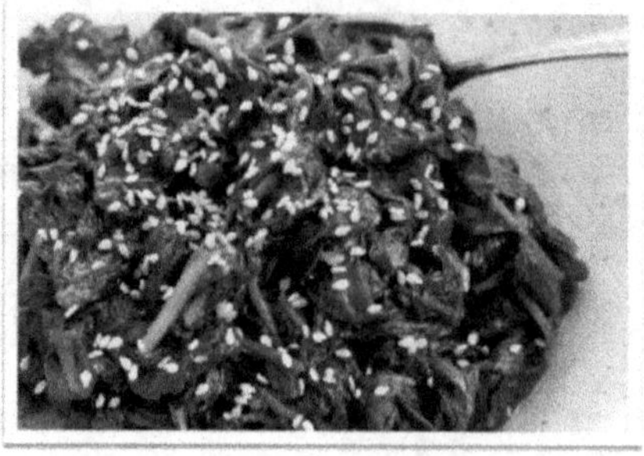

Preparation Time: 1 hr. 10 minutes

Cooking Time: 3 minutes

Servings: 04

Ingredients:

- 1 tablespoon toasted sesame oil
- ½ tablespoon soy sauce
- ½ teaspoon toasted sesame seeds, crushed
- ½ teaspoon rice vinegar
- ½ teaspoon golden caster sugar
- 1 garlic clove, grated
- 8 ounces spinach, stem ends trimmed

Directions:

1. Sauté spinach in a pan until it is wilted.
2. Whisk the sesame oil, garlic, sugar, vinegar, sesame seeds, soy sauce and black pepper together in a bowl.

3. Stir in spinach and mix well.
4. Cover and refrigerate for 1 hour.
5. Serve.

Nutrition: Calories: 677 Total Fat: 60g Carbs: 71g Net Carbs: 7g Fiber: 0g; Protein: 20g

PASTA & NOODLES

Stir Fry Noodles

Preparation Time: 10 minutes

Cooking Time: 8 minutes

Servings: 4

Ingredients:

- 1 cup broccoli, chopped
- 1 cup red bell pepper, chopped
- 1 cup mushrooms, chopped
- 1 large onion, chopped
- 1 batch Stir Fry Sauce, prepared
- Salt and black pepper, to taste
- 2 cups spaghetti, cooked
- 4 garlic cloves, minced
- 2 tablespoons sesame oil

Directions:

1. Heat sesame oil in a pan over medium heat and add garlic, onions, bell pepper, broccoli, mushrooms.

2. Sauté for about 5 minutes and add spaghetti noodles and stir fry sauce.
3. Mix well and cook for 3 more minutes.
4. Dish out in plates and serve to enjoy.

Nutrition: Calories: 567 Total fat: 48g Total carbs: 6g Fiber: 4g; Net carbs: 2g Sodium: 373mg Protein: 33g

Spicy Sweet Chili Veggie Noodles

Preparation Time: 10 minutes

Cooking Time: 7 minutes

Servings: 2

Ingredients:

- 1 head of broccoli, cut into bite sized florets
- 1 onion, finely sliced
- 1 tablespoon olive oil
- 1 courgette, halved
- 2 nests of whole-wheat noodles
- 150g mushrooms, sliced
- For Sauce
- 3 tablespoons soy sauce
- ¼ cup sweet chili sauce
- 1 teaspoon Sriracha
- 1 tablespoon peanut butter
- 2 tablespoons boiled water
- For Topping
- 2 teaspoons sesame seeds
- 2 teaspoons dried chili flakes

Directions:

1. Heat olive oil on medium heat in a saucepan and add onions.

2. Sauté for about 2 minutes and add broccoli, courgette and mushrooms.
3. Cook for about 5 minutes, stirring occasionally.
4. Whisk sweet chili sauce, soy sauce, Sriracha, water and peanut butter in a bowl.
5. Cook the noodles according to packet instructions and add to the vegetables.
6. Stir in the sauce and top with dried chili flakes and sesame seeds to serve.

Nutrition: Calories: 351 Total Fat: 27g Protein: 25g Total Carbs: 2g Fiber: 1g Net Carbs: 1g

Creamy Vegan Mushroom Pasta

Preparation Time: 10 minutes

Cooking Time: 30 minutes

Servings: 6

Ingredients:

- 2 cups frozen peas, thawed
- 3 tablespoons flour, unbleached
- 3 cups almond breeze, unsweetened
- 1 tablespoon nutritional yeast
- 1/3 cup fresh parsley, chopped, plus extra for garnish
- ¼ cup olive oil
- 1 pound pasta of choice
- 4 cloves garlic, minced
- 2/3 cup shallots, chopped
- 8 cups mixed mushrooms, sliced
- Salt and black pepper, to taste

Directions:

1. Take a bowl and boil pasta in salted water.
2. Heat olive oil in a pan over medium heat.
3. Add mushrooms, garlic, shallots and ½ tsp salt and cook for 15 minutes.

4. Sprinkle flour on the vegetables and stir for a minute while cooking.
5. Add almond beverage, stir constantly.
6. Let it simmer for 5 minutes and add pepper to it.
7. Cook for 3 more minutes and remove from heat.
8. Stir in nutritional yeast.
9. Add peas, salt, and pepper.
10. Cook for another minute and add
11. Add pasta to this sauce.
12. Garnish and serve!

Nutrition: Calories: 364 Total Fat: 28g Protein: 24g Total Carbs: 4g Fiber: 2g Net Carbs: 2g

Vegan Chinese Noodles

Preparation Time: 15 minutes

Cooking Time: 8 minutes

Servings: 4

Ingredients:

- 300 g mixed oriental mushrooms, such as oyster, shiitake and enoki, cleaned and sliced
- 200 g thin rice noodles, cooked according to packet instructions and drained
- 2 garlic cloves, minced
- 1 fresh red chili
- 200 g courgettes, sliced
- 6 spring onions, reserving the green part
- 1 teaspoon corn flour
- 1 tablespoon agave syrup
- 1 teaspoon sesame oil
- 100 g baby spinach, chopped
- Hot chili sauce, to serve
- 2(1-inch) pieces of ginger
- ½ bunch fresh coriander, chopped
- 4 tablespoons vegetable oil
- 2 tablespoons low-salt soy sauce
- ½ tablespoon rice wine

- 2 limes, to serve

Directions:

1. Heat sesame oil over high heat in a large wok and add the mushrooms.
2. Sauté for about 4 minutes and add garlic, chili, ginger, courgette, coriander stalks and the white part of the spring onions.
3. Sauté for about 3 minutes until softened and lightly golden.
4. Meanwhile, combine the corn flour and 2 tablespoons of water in a bowl.
5. Add soy sauce, agave syrup, sesame oil and rice wine to the corn flour mixture.
6. Put this mixture in the pan to the veggie mixture and cook for about 3 minutes until thickened.
7. Add the spinach and noodles and mix well.
8. Stir in the coriander leaves and top with lime wedges, hot chili sauce and reserved spring onions to serve.

Nutrition: Calories: 314 Total Fat: 22g Protein: 26g Total Carbs: 3g Fiber: 0.3g Net Carbs: 2.7g

Vegetable Penne Pasta

Preparation Time: 15 minutes

Cooking Time: 20 minutes

Servings: 6

Ingredients:

- ½ large onion, chopped
- 2 celery sticks, chopped
- ½ tablespoon ginger paste
- ½ cup green bell pepper
- 1½ tablespoons soy sauce
- ½ teaspoon parsley
- Salt and black pepper, to taste
- ½ pound penne pasta, cooked
- 2 large carrots, diced
- ½ small leek, chopped
- 1 tablespoon olive oil
- ½ teaspoon garlic paste
- ½ tablespoon Worcester sauce
- ½ teaspoon coriander
- 1 cup water

Directions:

1. Heat olive oil in a wok on medium heat and add onions, garlic and ginger paste.

2. Sauté for about 3 minutes and stir in all bell pepper, celery sticks, carrots and leek.
3. Sauté for about 5 minutes and add remaining ingredients except for pasta.
4. Cover the lid and cook for about 12 minutes.
5. Stir in the cooked pasta and dish out to serve warm.

Nutrition: Calories: 385 Total Fat: 29g Protein: 26g Total Carbs: 5g Fiber: 1g Net Carbs: 4g

Spaghetti in Spicy Tomato Sauce

Preparation Time: 15 minutes

Cooking Time: 40 minutes

Servings: 4

Ingredients:

- 1 pound dried spaghetti
- 1 red bell pepper, diced
- 4 garlic cloves, minced
- 1 teaspoon red pepper flakes, crushed
- 2 (14-ounce) cans diced tomatoes
- 1 (6-ounce) can tomato paste
- 2 teaspoons vegan sugar, granulated
- 2 tablespoons olive oil
- 1 medium onion, diced
- 1 cup dry red wine
- 1 teaspoon dried thyme
- ½ teaspoon fennel seed, crushed
- 1½ cups coconut milk, full-fat
- Salt and black pepper, to taste

Directions:

1. Boil water in a large pot and add pasta.
2. Cook according to the package directions and drain the pasta into a colander.

3. Dish out the pasta in a large serving bowl and add a dash of olive oil to prevent sticking.
4. Heat 2 tablespoons of olive oil over medium heat in a large pot and add garlic, onion and bell pepper.
5. Sauté for about 5 minutes and stir in the wine, thyme, fennel and red pepper flakes.
6. Allow to simmer on high heat for about 5 minutes until the liquid is reduced by about half.
7. Add diced tomatoes and tomato paste and allow to simmer for about 20 minutes, stirring occasionally.
8. Stir in the coconut milk and sugar and simmer for about 10 more minutes.
9. Season with salt and black pepper and pour the sauce over the pasta.
10. Toss to coat well and dish out in plates to serve.

Nutrition: Calories: 313 Total Fat: 25g Protein: 21g Total Carbs: 1g Fiber: 0g Net Carbs: 1g

20 Minutes Vegetarian Pasta

Preparation Time: 5 minutes

Cooking Time: 16 minutes

Servings: 4

Ingredients:

- 3 shallots, chopped
- ¼ teaspoon red pepper flakes
- ¼ cup vegan parmesan cheese
- 2 tablespoons olive oil
- 2 garlic cloves, minced
- 8-ounces spinach leaves
- 8-ounces linguine pasta
- 1 pinch salt
- 1 pinch black pepper

Directions:

1. Boil salted water in a large pot and add pasta.
2. Cook for about 6 minutes and drain the pasta in a colander.
3. Heat olive oil over medium heat in a large skillet and add the shallots.
4. Cook for about 5 minutes until soft and caramelized and stir in the spinach, garlic, red pepper flakes, salt and black pepper.

5. Cook for about 5 minutes and add pasta and 2 ladles of pasta water.
6. Stir in the parmesan cheese and dish out in a bowl to serve.

Nutrition: Calories: 284 Total Fat: 18g Protein: 29g Total Carbs: 1.5g Fiber: 0g Net Carbs: 1.5g

Creamy Vegan Pumpkin Pasta

Preparation Time: 15 minutes

Cooking Time: 5 minutes

Servings: 6

Ingredients:

- 1 tablespoon olive oil
- 1 cup raw cashews, soaked in water 4-8 hours, drained and rinsed
- 12 ounces dried penne pasta
- 1 cup pumpkin puree, canned
- 1 cup almond milk, plus more as needed
- 3 garlic cloves
- ¼ teaspoon ground nutmeg
- Fresh parsley, for garnish
- 1 tablespoon lemon juice
- ¾ teaspoon salt
- 1 tablespoon fresh sage, chopped

Directions:

1. Boil salted water in a large pot and add pasta.
2. Cook according to the package directions and drain the pasta into a colander.
3. Dish out the pasta in a large serving bowl and add a dash of olive oil to prevent sticking.

4. Put the pumpkin, cashews, milk, lemon juice, garlic, salt and nutmeg into the food processor and blend until smooth.
5. Stir in the sauce and sage over the pasta and toss to coat well.
6. Garnish with fresh parsley and dish out to serve hot.

NUTRITION: Calories: 431 Total Fat: 31g Protein: 35g Total Carbs: 3g Fiber: 0.5g Net Carbs: 2.5g

Loaded Creamy Vegan Pesto Pasta

Preparation Time: 15 minutes

Cooking Time: 10 minutes

Servings: 6

Ingredients:

- ¼ onion, finely chopped
- 8 romaine lettuce leaves
- 1 celery stalk, thinly sliced
- ½ cup blue cheese, crumbled
- 1 tablespoon olive oil, plus a dash
- 1 cup almond milk, unflavored and unsweetened
- ½ cup vegan pesto
- 1 cup chickpeas, cooked
- 1 cup fresh arugula, packed
- 2 tablespoons lemon juice
- Salt and black pepper, to taste
- 6-ounces orecchiette pasta, dried
- 1 cup full-fat coconut milk
- 2 tablespoons whole wheat flour
- 1½ cups cherry tomatoes, halved
- ½ cup Kalamata olives, halved

- Red pepper flakes, to taste

Directions:

1. Boil salted water in a large pot and add pasta.
2. Cook according to the package directions and drain the pasta into a colander.
3. Dish out the pasta in a large serving bowl and add a dash of olive oil to prevent sticking.
4. Put olive oil over medium heat in a large pot and whisk in the flour.
5. Cook for about 4 minutes, until the mixture begins to smell nutty and stir in the coconut milk and almond milk.
6. Let the sauce simmer for about 1 minute and add the chickpeas, olives and arugula.
7. Stir well and season with lemon juice, red pepper flakes, and salt and black pepper.
8. Dish out into plates and serve hot.

Nutrition: Calories: 220 Total Fat: 10g Protein: 31g Total Carbs: 1.5g Fiber: 0.5g Net Carbs: 1g

Creamy Vegan Spinach Pasta

Preparation Time: 20 minutes

Cooking Time: 5 minutes

Servings: 4

Ingredients:

- 1 cup raw cashews, soaked in water for 8 hours
- 2 tablespoons lemon juice
- 1 tablespoon olive oil
- 1½ cups vegetable broth
- 2 tablespoons fresh dill, chopped
- Red pepper flakes, to taste
- 10 ounces dried fusilli
- ½ cup almond milk, unflavored and unsweetened
- 2 tablespoons white miso paste
- 4 garlic cloves, divided
- 8-ounces fresh spinach, finely chopped
- ¼ cup scallions, chopped
- Salt and black pepper, to taste

Directions:

1. Boil salted water in a large pot and add pasta.
2. Cook according to the package directions and drain the pasta into a colander.

3. Dish out the pasta in a large serving bowl and add a dash of olive oil to prevent sticking.
4. Put the cashews, milk, miso, lemon juice, and 1 garlic clove into the food processor and blend until smooth.
5. Put olive oil over medium heat in a large pot and add the remaining 3 cloves of garlic.
6. Sauté for about 1 minute and stir in the spinach and broth.
7. Raise the heat and allow to simmer for about 4 minutes until the spinach is bright green and wilted.
8. Stir in the pasta and cashew mixture and season with salt and black pepper.
9. Top with scallions and dill and dish out into plates to serve.

Nutrition: Calories: 94 Total Fat: 10g Protein: 0g Total Carbs: 1g Fiber: 0.3g Net Carbs: 0.7g

Vegan Bake Pasta with Bolognese Sauce and Cashew Cream

Preparation Time: 1 hour 10 minutes

Cooking Time: 20 minutes

Servings: 8

Ingredients:

For the Pasta:

- 1 packet penne pasta

For the Bolognese Sauce:

- 1 tablespoon soy sauce
- 1 small can lentils
- 1 tablespoon brown sugar
- ½ cup tomato paste
- 1 teaspoon garlic, crushed
- 1 tablespoon olive oil
- 2 tomatoes, chopped
- 1 onion, chopped
- 2 cups mushrooms, sliced
- Salt, to taste
- Pepper, to taste
- For the Cashew Cream:
- 1 cup raw cashews

- ½ lemon, squeezed
- ½ teaspoon salt
- ½ cup water
- For the White Sauce:
- 1 teaspoon black pepper
- 1 teaspoon Dijon mustard
- ¼ cup nutritional yeast
- Sea salt, as required
- 2 cups coconut milk
- 3 tablespoons vegan butter
- 2 tablespoons all-purpose flour
- 1/3 cup vegetable broth

Directions:

1. Take a pot and boil water, add pasta to it, boil for 3 minutes and set aside.
2. Fry onion and garlic, mushroom in olive oil and add soy sauce to it.
3. Add in sugar tomato paste, lentils, and canned tomato to it and let it simmer, Bolognese sauce is prepared.
4. Season it with salt and black pepper.
5. Add the lemon juice, cashews, water and salt to the blender, blend for 2 minutes.

6. Add this to the sauce you have prepared and stir pasta in it.
7. Melt the vegan butter in a saucepan, add in the flour and stir.
8. Add vegetable stock and coconut milk to it and whisk well.
9. Stir continuously and let it boil for about 5 minutes, then remove from heat.
10. Add Dijon mustard, nutritional yeast, black pepper, and sea salt.
11. Preheat the oven to 430 degrees F.
12. Prepare rectangular oven-safe dish by placing pasta and Bolognese sauce to it.
13. Pour the white sauce on it and bake for a time period of 20-25 minutes.

Nutrition: Calories: 314 Total Fat: 20g Protein: 31g Total Carbs: 2.5g Fiber: 0.8g Net Carbs: 1.7g

Asian Veggie Noodles

Preparation Time: 10 minutes

Cooking Time: 20 minutes

Servings: 4

Ingredients:

- ½ cup peas
- 1 teaspoon rice vinegar
- 3 carrots, chopped
- 1 small packet vermicelli
- 3 tablespoons sesame oil
- 1 red pepper, chopped in small cubes
- 1 can baby corn
- 1 clove garlic, chopped
- 2 tablespoons soy sauce
- 1 teaspoon ginger powder
- ½ teaspoon curry powder
- Salt and black pepper, to taste

Directions:

1. Take a bowl and add ginger powder, vinegar, soy sauce, curry powder, and a pinch of salt to it.
2. Cook the noodles according to the instructions and drain them.

3. Heat the sesame oil and cook vegetables in it for 10 minutes on medium heat.
4. Add noodles to it and cook for 3 more minutes.
5. Remove from heat and serve to enjoy.

Nutrition: Calories: 329 Total Fat: 25g Protein: 20g Total Carbs: 6g Fiber: 1g Net Carbs: 5g

5 Ingredients Pasta

Preparation Time: 15 minutes

Cooking Time: 25 minutes

Servings: 5

Ingredients:

- 1 (25 oz.) jar marinara sauce
- Olive oil, as needed
- 1 pound dry vegan pasta
- 1 pound assorted vegetables, like red onion, zucchini and tomatoes
- ¼ cup prepared hummus
- Salt, to taste

Directions:

1. Preheat the oven to 400 degrees F and grease a large baking sheet.
2. Arrange the vegetables in a single layer on the baking sheet and sprinkle with olive oil and salt.
3. Transfer into the oven and roast the vegetables for about 15 minutes.
4. Boil salted water in a large pot and cook the pasta according to the package directions.
5. Drain the water when the pasta is tender and put the pasta in a colander.

6. Mix together the marinara sauce and hummus in a large pot to make a creamy sauce.
7. Stir in the cooked vegetables and pasta to the sauce and toss to coat well.
8. Dish out in a bowl and serve warm.

Nutrition: Calories: 415 Total Fat: 29g Protein: 33g Total Carbs: 5.5g Fiber: 2g Net Carbs: 3.5g

SMOOTHIES AND BEVERAGES

Kale Smoothie

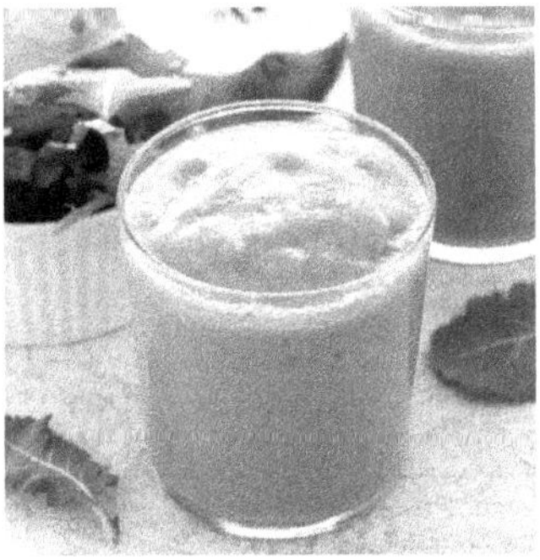

Preparation Time: 5 minutes

Cooking Time: 0 minutes

Servings: 2

Ingredients:

- 2 cups chopped kale leaves
- 1 banana, peeled
- 1 cup frozen strawberries
- 1 cup unsweetened almond milk
- 4 Medjool dates, pitted and chopped

Directions:

1. Put all the ingredients in a food processor, then blitz until glossy and smooth.

2. Serve immediately or chill in the refrigerator for an hour before serving.

Nutrition: Calories: 663 Fat: 10.0g Carbs: 142.5g Fiber: 19.0g Protein: 17.4g

Hot Tropical Smoothie

Preparation Time: 5 minutes

Cooking Time: 0 minutes

Servings: 4

Ingredients:

- 1 cup frozen mango chunks
- 1 cup frozen pineapple chunks
- 1 small tangerine, peeled and pitted
- 2 cups spinach leaves
- 1 cup coconut water
- ¼ teaspoon cayenne pepper, optional

Directions:

1. Add all the ingredients in a food processor, then blitz until the mixture is smooth and combine well.
2. Serve immediately or chill in the refrigerator for an hour before serving.

Nutrition: Calories: 283 Fat: 1.9g Carbs: 67.9g Fiber: 10.4g Protein: 6.4g

Berry Smoothie

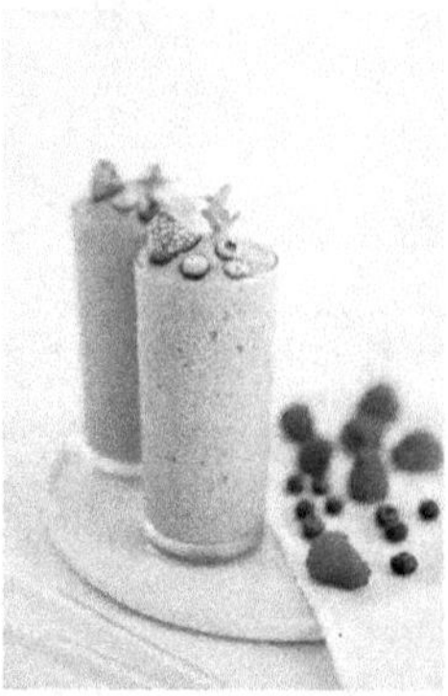

Preparation Time: 5 minutes

Cooking Time: 0 minutes

Servings: 4

Ingredients:

- 1 cup berry mix (strawberries, blueberries, and cranberries)
- 4 Medjool dates, pitted and chopped
- 1½ cups unsweetened almond milk, plus more as needed

Directions:

1. Add all the ingredients in a blender, then process until the mixture is smooth and well mixed.
2. Serve immediately or chill in the refrigerator for an hour before serving.

Nutrition: Calories: 473 Fat: 4.0g Carbs: 103.7g Fiber: 9.7g Protein: 14.8g

Cranberry and Banana Smoothie

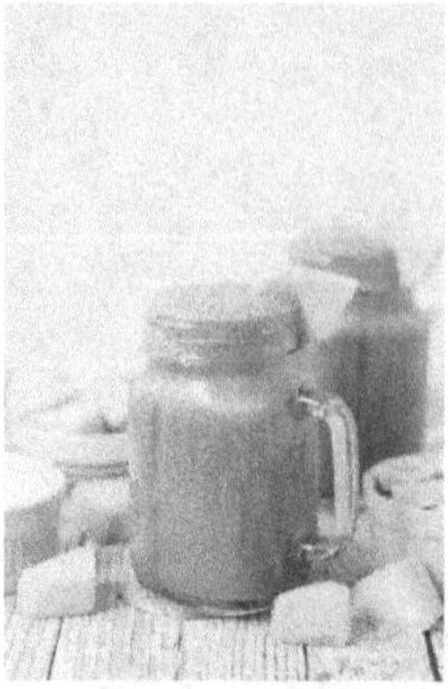

Preparation Time: 5 minutes

Cooking Time: 0 minutes

Servings: 4

- 1 cup frozen cranberries
- 1 large banana, peeled
- 4 Medjool dates, pitted and chopped
- 1½ cups unsweetened almond milk

Directions:

1. Add all the ingredients in a food processor, then process until the mixture is glossy and well mixed.
2. Serve immediately or chill in the refrigerator for an hour before serving.

Nutrition: Calories: 616 Fat: 8.0g Carbs: 132.8g Fiber: 14.6g Protein: 15.7g

Pumpkin Smoothie

Preparation Time: 5 minutes

Cooking Time: 0 minutes

Servings: 5

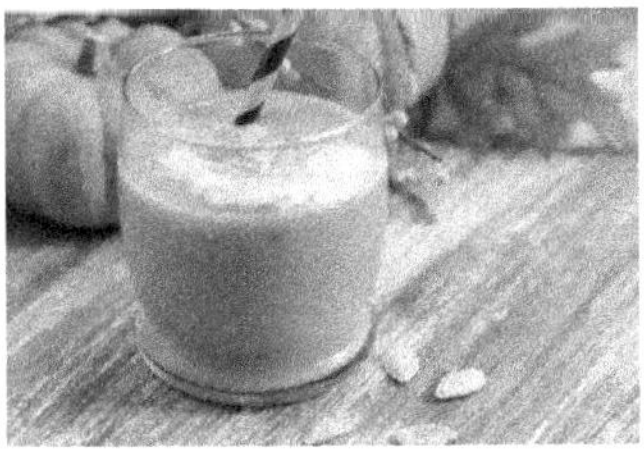

Ingredients:

- ½ cup pumpkin purée
- 4 Medjool dates, pitted and chopped
- 1 cup unsweetened almond milk
- ¼ teaspoon vanilla extract
- ¼ teaspoon ground cinnamon
- ½ cup ice
- Pinch ground nutmeg

Directions:

1. Add all the ingredients in a blender, then process until the mixture is glossy and well mixed.
2. Serve immediately.

Nutrition: Calories: 417 Fat: 3.0g Carbs: 94.9g Fiber: 10.4g Protein: 11.4g

Super Smoothie

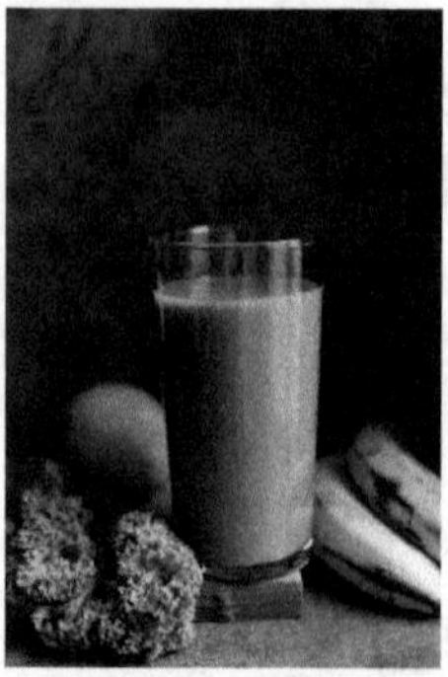

Preparation Time: 5 minutes

Cooking Time: 0 minutes

Servings: 4

Ingredients:

- 1 banana, peeled
- 1 cup chopped mango
- 1 cup raspberries
- ¼ cup rolled oats
- 1 carrot, peeled
- 1 cup chopped fresh kale
- 2 tablespoons chopped fresh parsley
- 1 tablespoon flaxseeds
- 1 tablespoon grated fresh ginger
- ½ cup unsweetened soy milk
- 1 cup water

Directions:

1. Put all the ingredients in a food processor, then blitz until glossy and smooth.
2. Serve immediately or chill in the refrigerator for an hour before serving.

Nutrition: Calories: 550 Fat: 39.0g Carbs: 31.0g Fiber: 15.0g Protein: 13.0g

Kiwi and Strawberry Smoothie

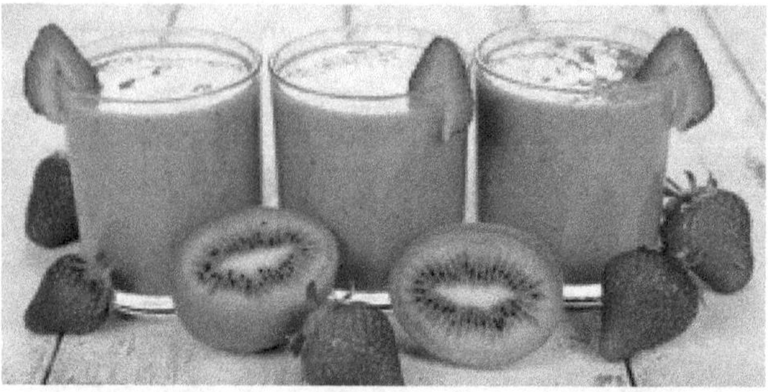

Preparation Time: 5 minutes

Cooking Time: 0 minutes

Servings: 3

Ingredients:

- 1 kiwi, peeled
- 5 medium strawberries
- ½ frozen banana
- 1 cup unsweetened almond milk
- 2 tablespoons hemp seeds
- 2 tablespoons peanut butter
- 1 to 2 teaspoons maple syrup
- ½ cup spinach leaves
- Handful broccoli sprouts

Directions:

1. Put all the ingredients in a food processor, then blitz until creamy and smooth.

2. Serve immediately or chill in the refrigerator for an hour before serving.

Nutrition: Calories: 562 Fat: 28.6g Carbs: 63.6g Fiber: 15.1g Protein: 23.3g

Banana and Chai Chia Smoothie

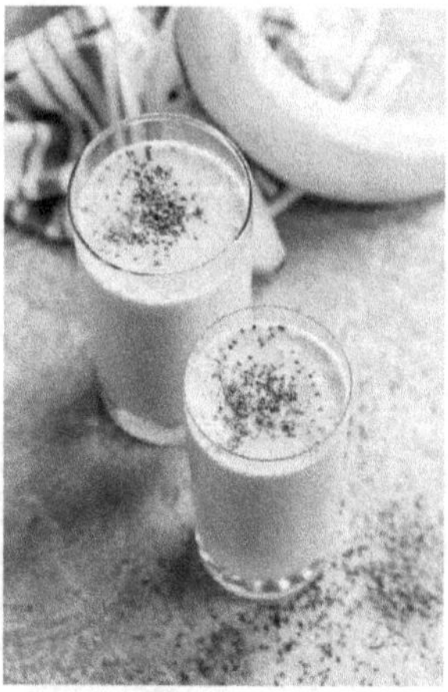

Preparation Time: 5 minutes

Cooking Time: 0 minutes

Servings: 3

Ingredients:

- 1 banana
- 1 cup alfalfa sprouts
- 1 tablespoon chia seeds
- ½ cup unsweetened coconut milk
- 1 to 2 soft Medjool dates, pitted
- ¼ teaspoon ground cinnamon
- 1 tablespoon grated fresh ginger
- 1 cup water
- Pinch ground cardamom

Directions:

1. Add all the ingredients in a blender, then process until the mixture is smooth and creamy. Add water or coconut milk if necessary.
2. Serve immediately.

Nutrition: Calories: 477 Fat: 41.0g Carbs: 31.0g Fiber: 14.0g Protein: 8.0g

Chocolate and Peanut Butter Smoothie

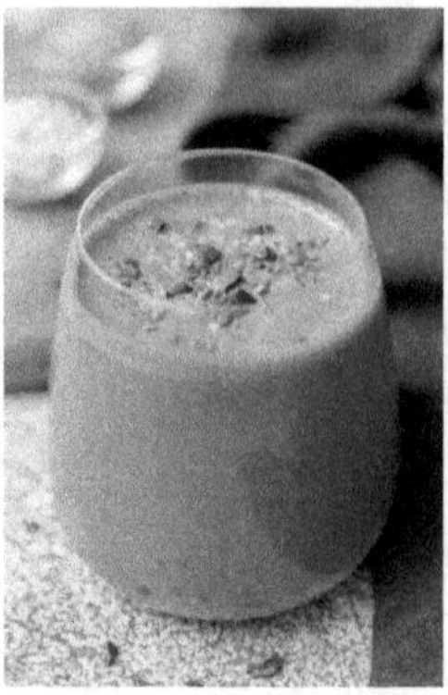

Preparation Time: 5 minutes

Cooking Time: 0 minutes

Servings: 4

Ingredients:

- 1 tablespoon unsweetened cocoa powder
- 1 tablespoon peanut butter
- 1 banana
- 1 teaspoon maca powder
- ½ cup unsweetened soy milk
- ¼ cup rolled oats
- 1 tablespoon flaxseeds
- 1 tablespoon maple syrup
- 1 cup water

Directions:

1. Add all the ingredients in a blender, then process until the mixture is smooth and creamy. Add water or soy milk if necessary.
2. Serve immediately.

Nutrition: Calories: 474 Fat: 16.0g Carbs: 27.0g Fiber: 18.0g Protein: 13.0g

Golden Milk

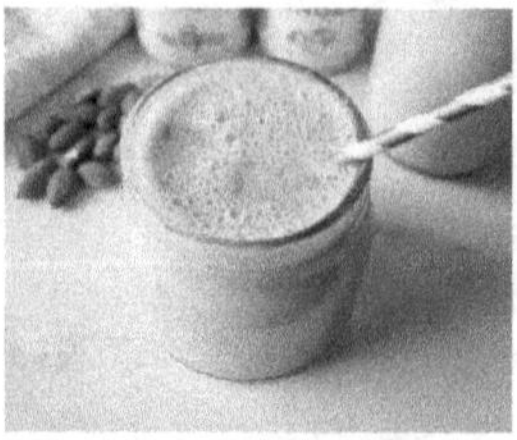

Preparation Time: 5 minutes

Cooking Time: 0 minutes

Servings: 4

Ingredients:

- ¼ teaspoon ground cinnamon
- ½ teaspoon ground turmeric
- ½ teaspoon grated fresh ginger
- 1 teaspoon maple syrup
- 1 cup unsweetened coconut milk
- Ground black pepper, to taste
- 2 tablespoon water

Directions:

1. Combine all the ingredients in a saucepan. Stir to mix well.
2. Heat over medium heat for 5 minutes. Keep stirring during the heating.

3. Allow to cool for 5 minutes, then pour the mixture in a blender. Pulse until creamy and smooth. Serve immediately.

Nutrition: Calories: 577 Fat: 57.3g Carbs: 19.7g Fiber: 6.1g Protein: 5.7g

Mango Agua Fresca

Preparation Time: 5 minutes

Cooking Time: 0 minutes

Servings: 2

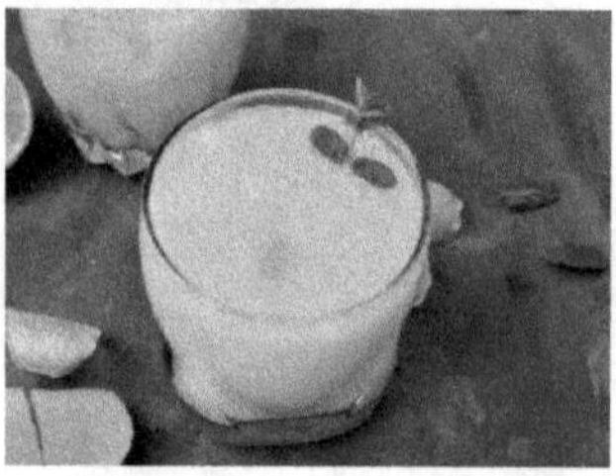

Ingredients:

- 2 fresh mangoes, diced
- 1½ cups water
- 1 teaspoon fresh lime juice
- Maple syrup, to taste
- 2 cups ice
- 2 slices fresh lime, for garnish
- 2 fresh mint sprigs, for garnish

Directions:

1. Put the mangoes, lime juice, maple syrup, and water in a blender. Process until creamy and smooth.

2. Divide the beverage into two glasses, then garnish each glass with ice, lime slice, and mint sprig before serving.

Nutrition: Calories: 230 Fat: 1.3g Carbs: 57.7g Fiber: 5.4g Protein: 2.8g

Light Ginger Tea

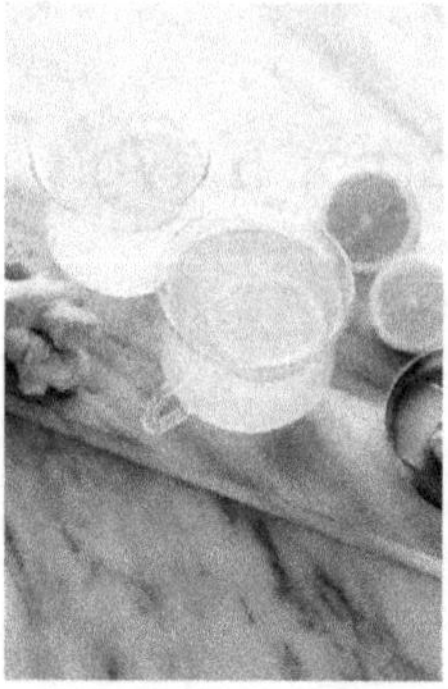

Preparation Time: 5 minutes

Cooking Time: 10 to 15 minutes

Servings: 2

Ingredients:

- 1 small ginger knob, sliced into four 1-inch chunks
- 4 cups water
- Juice of 1 large lemon
- Maple syrup, to taste

Directions:

1. Add the ginger knob and water in a saucepan, then simmer over medium heat for 10 to 15 minutes.

2. Turn off the heat, then mix in the lemon juice. Strain the liquid to remove the ginger, then fold in the maple syrup and serve.

Nutrition: Calories: 32 Fat: 0.1g Carbs: 8.6g Fiber: 0.1g Protein: 0.1g

Classic Switchel

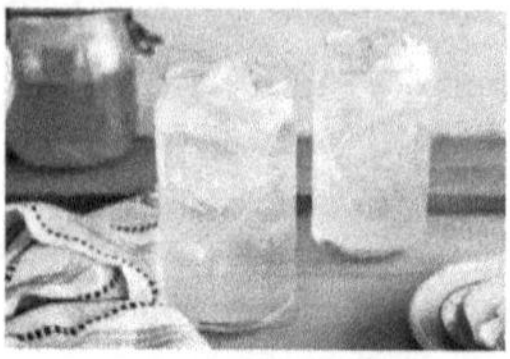

Preparation Time: 5 minutes

Cooking Time: 0 minutes

Servings: 4

Ingredients:

- 1-inch piece ginger, minced
- 2 tablespoons apple cider vinegar
- 2 tablespoons maple syrup
- 4 cups water
- ¼ teaspoon sea salt, optional

Directions:

1. Combine all the ingredients in a glass. Stir to mix well.
2. Serve immediately or chill in the refrigerator for an hour before serving.

Nutrition: Calories: 110 Fat: 0g Carbs: 28.0g Fiber: 0g Protein: 0g

Lime and Cucumber Electrolyte Drink

Preparation Time: 5 minutes

Cooking Time: 0 minutes

Servings: 4

Ingredients:

- ¼ cup chopped cucumber
- 1 tablespoon fresh lime juice
- 1 tablespoon apple cider vinegar
- 2 tablespoons maple syrup
- ¼ teaspoon sea salt, optional
- 4 cups water

Directions:

1. Combine all the ingredients in a glass. Stir to mix well.
2. Refrigerate overnight before serving.

Nutrition: Calories: 114 Fat: 0.1g Carbs: 28.9g Fiber: 0.3g Protein: 0.3g

Easy and Fresh Mango Madness

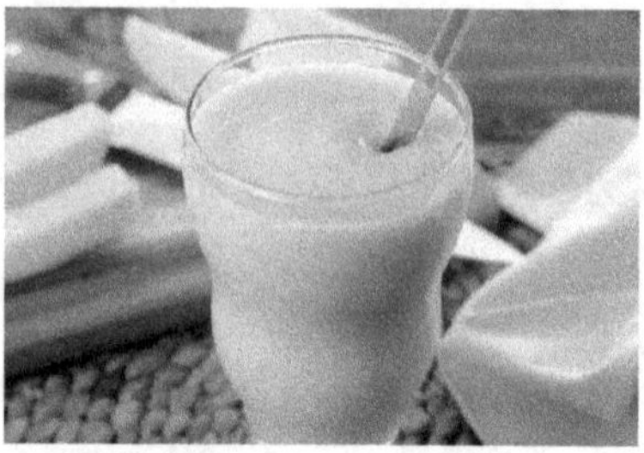

Preparation Time: 5 minutes

Cooking Time: 0 minutes

Servings: 4

Ingredients:

- 1 cup chopped mango
- 1 cup chopped peach
- 1 banana
- 1 cup strawberries
- 1 carrot, peeled and chopped
- 1 cup water

Directions:

1. Put all the ingredients in a food processor, then blitz until glossy and smooth.
2. Serve immediately or chill in the refrigerator for an hour before serving.

Nutrition: Calories: 376 Fat: 22.0g Carbs: 19.0g Fiber: 14.0g Protein: 5.0g

Simple Date Shake

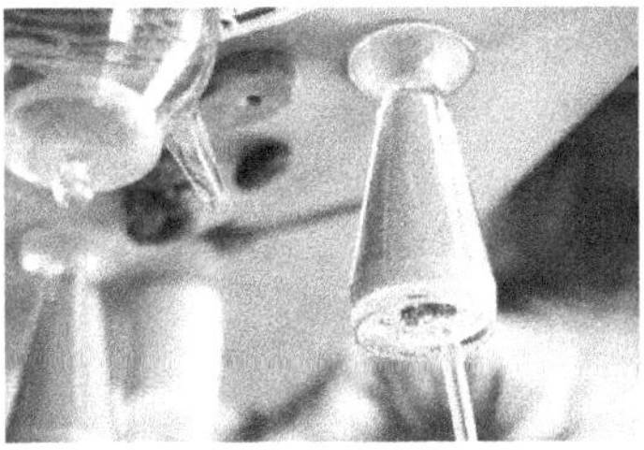

Preparation Time: 10 minutes

Cooking Time: 0 minutes

Servings: 2

Ingredients:

- 5 Medjool dates, pitted, soaked in boiling water for 5 minutes
- ¾ cup unsweetened coconut milk
- 1 teaspoon vanilla extract
- ½ teaspoon fresh lemon juice
- ¼ teaspoon sea salt, optional
- 1½ cups ice

Directions:

1. Put all the ingredients in a food processor, then blitz until it has a milkshake and smooth texture.
2. Serve immediately.

Nutrition: Calories: 380 Fat: 21.6g Carbs: 50.3g Fiber: 6.0g Protein: 3.2g

Beet and Clementine Protein Smoothie

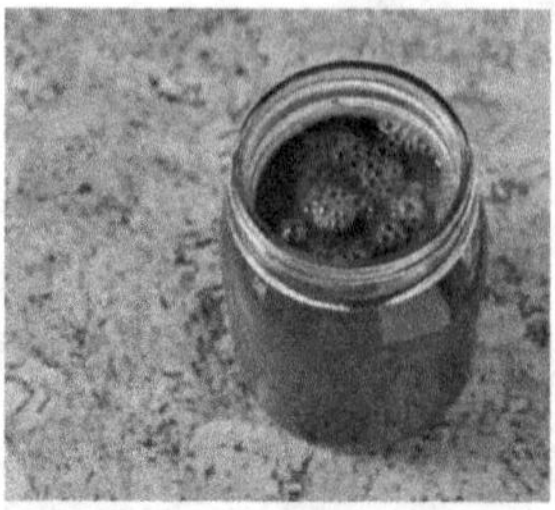

Preparation Time: 10 minutes

Cooking Time: 0 minutes

Servings: 3

Ingredients:

- 1 small beet, peeled and chopped
- 1 clementine, peeled and broken into segments
- ½ ripe banana
- ½ cup raspberries
- 1 tablespoon chia seeds
- 2 tablespoons almond butter
- ¼ teaspoon vanilla extract
- 1 cup unsweetened almond milk
- 1/8 teaspoon fine sea salt, optional

Directions:

1. Combine all the ingredients in a food processor, then pulse on high for 2 minutes or until glossy and creamy.
2. Refrigerate for an hour and serve chilled.

Nutrition: **Calories: 526 Fat: 25.4g Carbs: 61.9g Fiber: 17.3g Protein: 20.6g**

Conclusion

Vegan recipes do not need to be boring. There are so many different combinations of veggies, fruits, whole grains, beans, seeds, and nuts that you will be able to make unique meal plans for many months. These recipes contain the instructions along with the necessary ingredients and nutritional information.

If you ever come across someone complaining that they can't follow the plant-based diet because it's expensive, hard to cater for, lacking in variety, or tasteless, feel free to have them take a look at this book. In no time, you'll have another companion walking beside you on this road to healthier eating and better living.

Although healthy, many people are still hesitant to give vegan food a try. They mistakenly believe that these would be boring, tasteless, and complicated to make. This is the farthest thing from the truth.

Fruits and vegetables are organically delicious, fragrant, and vibrantly colored. If you add herbs, mushrooms, and nuts to the mix, dishes will always come out packed full of flavor it only takes a bit of effort and time to prepare great-tasting vegan meals for your family.

How easy was that? Don't we all want a seamless and easy way to cook like this?

I believe cooking is taking a better turn and the days, when we needed so many ingredients to provide a decent meal, were gone. Now, with easy tweaks, we can make delicious, quick, and easy meals. Most importantly, we get to save a bunch of cash on groceries.

I am grateful for downloading this book and taking the time to read it. I know that you have learned a lot and you had a great time reading it. Writing books is the best way to share the skills I have with your and the best tips too.

I know that there are many books and choosing my book is amazing. I am thankful that you stopped and took time to decide. You made a great decision and I am sure that you enjoyed it.

I will be even happier if you will add some comments. Feedbacks helped by growing and they still do. They help me to choose better content and new ideas. So, maybe your feedback can trigger an idea for my next book.

Hopefully, this book has helped you understand that vegetarian recipes and diet can improve your life, not only by improving your health and helping you lose weight, but also by saving you money and time. I sincerely hope that the recipes provided in this book have proven to be quick, easy, and delicious, and have provided you with enough variety to keep your taste buds interested and curious.

I hope you enjoyed reading about my book!

CPSIA information can be obtained
at www.ICGtesting.com
Printed in the USA
LVHW081813010621
689062LV00015B/1729

9 781803 040790